Leg Ulcers

A Beginner's Quick Start Guide to Managing Leg Ulcers Through Diet and Other Natural Methods, With Sample Recipes and a 7-Day Meal Plan

mf

copyright © 2022 Patrick Marshwell

All rights reserved No part of this book may be reproduced, or stored in a retrieval system, or transmitted in any form or by any means, electronic, mechanical, photocopying, recording, or otherwise, without express written permission of the publisher.

Disclaimer

By reading this disclaimer, you are accepting the terms of the disclaimer in full. If you disagree with this disclaimer, please do not read the guide.

All of the content within this guide is provided for informational and educational purposes only, and should not be accepted as independent medical or other professional advice. The author is not a doctor, physician, nurse, mental health provider, or registered nutritionist/dietician. Therefore, using and reading this guide does not establish any form of a physician-patient relationship.

Always consult with a physician or another qualified health provider with any issues or questions you might have regarding any sort of medical condition. Do not ever disregard any qualified professional medical advice or delay seeking that advice because of anything you have read in this guide. The information in this guide is not intended to be any sort of medical advice and should not be used in lieu of any medical advice by a licensed and qualified medical professional.

The information in this guide has been compiled from a variety of known sources. However, the author cannot attest to or guarantee the accuracy of each source and thus should not be held liable for any errors or omissions.

You acknowledge that the publisher of this guide will not be held liable for any loss or damage of any kind incurred as a result of this guide or the reliance on any information provided within this guide. You acknowledge and agree that you assume all risk and responsibility for any action you undertake in response to the information in this guide.

Using this guide does not guarantee any particular result (e.g., weight loss or a cure). By reading this guide, you acknowledge that there are no guarantees to any specific outcome or results you can expect.

All product names, diet plans, or names used in this guide are for identification purposes only and are the property of their respective owners. The use of these names does not imply endorsement. All other trademarks cited herein are the property of their respective owners.

Where applicable, this guide is not intended to be a substitute for the original work of this diet plan and is, at most, a supplement to the original work for this diet plan and never a direct substitute. This guide is a personal expression of the facts of that diet plan.

Where applicable, persons shown in the cover images are stock photography models and the publisher has obtained the rights to use the images through license agreements with third-party stock image companies.

Table of Contents

Introduction	**7**
What Are Leg Ulcers?	**9**
What Causes Leg Ulcers?	10
What Are the Symptoms of Leg Ulcers?	**13**
When Should I See a Doctor?	15
How Are Leg Ulcers Diagnosed?	15
Leg Ulcers Risk Factors	16
What Are the Complications of Leg Ulcers?	18
How Can You Prevent Leg Ulcers?	**20**
Different Treatments for Leg Ulcers	**22**
Traditional Treatments	22
Natural Treatments	23
Ways to Manage Leg Ulcers	**25**
Home Therapy	25
Diet	26
7-Day Sample Meal Plan	30
Sample Recipes	**32**
No-Fuss Tuna Casserole	33
Tangy Lemon Fish	34
Vietnamese Early Rush Baguette	36
Macrobiotic Apple and Oats Porridge	38
Vegan Tiramisu	39
Nut Truffle	41
Blackened Shrimp	42
Grilled Tuna	43
Chicken Pot Pie	44
Apple in Pork Chops	47
Kale Fried Rice	49
Grilled Eggplant	51

Low FODMAP Burger	52
Roasted Chicken Thighs	53
Steamed Cauliflower and Curried Shrimp	54
Conclusion	**56**
FAQ	**57**
Key Takeaways	58
References and Helpful Links	**60**

Introduction

Leg ulcers are open wounds that can occur on the legs. Leg ulcers are a common problem, especially among the elderly. They can be caused by several factors, including circulatory problems and diabetes.

If left untreated, they can lead to serious health complications. Although they can be painful, fortunately, there are treatments available that can help heal leg ulcers and prevent them from returning.

Leg ulcers can be a real pain, both literally and figuratively. They are often slow to heal and can be quite uncomfortable. But they don't have to be a lifelong burden. There are many things you can do to help manage them naturally, from simple home remedies to changes in your diet. This guide will outline some of the best ways to do that naturally, through diet and home remedies.

In this beginner's quick start guide, we'll cover:

- All about leg ulcers
- Causes and symptoms of leg ulcers

- Leg ulcer diagnosis and risk factors
- Ways to manage and treat leg ulcers
- The right diet for leg ulcer

So, read on to learn more about leg ulcers, how to heal them naturally, and what dietary changes can help.

What Are Leg Ulcers?

Leg ulcers are open wounds that can occur on the legs. They are usually slow to heal and can be quite painful. The most common type of leg ulcer is a venous ulcer, which occurs when the veins in your legs are not working properly and allow blood to pool. This can cause the skin to thin and break down, leading to an ulcer.

Venous ulcers are the most common type of leg ulcer, accounting for about 80% of all cases. However, there are other types of leg ulcers as well, including:

Arterial ulcers are less common than venous ulcers and are caused by reduced blood flow to the legs. These ulcers usually occur on the toes or feet and are more likely to be painful than venous ulcers.

Neuropathic ulcers are caused by nerve damage, which can be due to diabetes or other conditions. These ulcers usually occur on the bottom of the feet and can be very painful.

Pressure ulcers are caused by sustained pressure on an area of the skin, which can occur when you are bedridden or have limited mobility. These ulcers usually occur on bony areas of the body, such as the heels or hips.

Infectious ulcers are caused by bacteria, viruses, or fungi. They can occur anywhere on the body and can be quite painful.

Mixed ulcers are a combination of two or more of the above types of leg ulcers.

What Causes Leg Ulcers?

Several different factors can contribute to the development of leg ulcers. The most common cause is venous insufficiency, which occurs when the veins in your legs are not working properly and allow blood to pool. This can be due to several different factors, including:

Venous valves

The veins in your legs have valves that open and close to ensure that blood flows in the correct direction. When these valves are damaged or not functioning properly, blood can pool in your legs, leading to venous insufficiency.

Obstruction

Obstruction of the veins can occur due to several different things, including blood clots, tumors, or inflammation. This can cause venous insufficiency and lead to leg ulcers.

Trauma

Injury to the veins can occur due to surgery, trauma, or radiation therapy. This can damage the valves in your veins and lead to venous insufficiency.

Aging

As you age, the veins in your legs can become less elastic and more likely to develop valves that are damaged or not functioning properly. This can lead to venous insufficiency and leg ulcers.

Obesity

Obesity can put extra pressure on the veins in your legs and make them more likely to develop valves that are damaged or not functioning properly. This can lead to venous insufficiency and leg ulcers.

Pregnancy

Pregnancy can cause the veins in your legs to enlarge and put extra pressure on the valves. This can lead to venous insufficiency and leg ulcers.

Sedentary lifestyle

A sedentary lifestyle can cause the veins in your legs to become more sluggish and more likely to develop valves that are damaged or not functioning properly. This can lead to venous insufficiency and leg ulcers.

Other causes of leg ulcers include arterial insufficiency, neuropathy, pressure ulcers, and infection.

What Are the Symptoms of Leg Ulcers?

The most common symptom of a leg ulcer is a break in the skin that does not heal. Other symptoms can include:

Pain

One symptom of a leg ulcer is pain. Leg ulcers can be quite painful, especially when they are located on bony areas of the foot or ankle, or when the ulcer is infected. The pain may worsen when the ulcer is touched or when pressure is applied to the area. In some cases, the pain may be so severe that it interferes with daily activities.

Swelling

Leg ulcers are often characterized by swelling in the affected area. This can be caused by a buildup of fluid in the tissue, known as edema. Edema can occur for a variety of reasons, including heart failure, kidney disease, and lymphatic disorders.

Crusting

One symptom of a leg ulcer is crusting. This occurs when the ulcer forms a hard, dry layer on the surface of the skin. Crusting can make the ulcer difficult to heal, as it can prevent new skin cells from growing. In addition, crusting can make the ulcer more painful, as the hard surface can rub against the surrounding skin. If you have an ulcer that is crusting, it is important to seek medical treatment, as this can help to prevent further damage to the skin.

Bleeding

One common symptom of a leg ulcer is bleeding. While any kind of cut or scrape has the potential to bleed, leg ulcers are more likely to do so because they often occur on an artery. When an ulcer bleeds, it can cause the skin around the wound to turn red or purple. In some cases, the bleeding may be severe enough to require medical attention.

Odor

One symptom of a leg ulcer is an unpleasant odor. This is usually caused by an infection, which can occur when the open sore is exposed to bacteria. The bacteria cause the wound to emit a foul smell.

Fever

Leg ulcers are sores that develop on the legs, often as a result of an infection. They can range in severity from small, superficial sores to large, deep wounds. Leg ulcers are often painful and can make it difficult to walk or stand. Infected leg ulcers can sometimes cause a fever.

When Should I See a Doctor?

You should see a doctor if you have any of the following symptoms:

- A sore on your leg that does not heal within two weeks
- Redness, swelling, or drainage from a leg ulcer
- Fever, chills, or body aches
- Leg pain that interferes with daily activities
- Changes in skin color around a leg ulcer
- A leg ulcer that gets worse despite home treatment

How Are Leg Ulcers Diagnosed?

Leg ulcers are usually diagnosed based on their appearance. Your doctor will likely ask about your medical history and do a physical exam. They may also order tests to look for underlying conditions that could be causing your leg ulcers. These tests may include:

- Blood tests can help to look for underlying conditions that could be causing your leg ulcers, such as diabetes or an infection.
- Imaging tests, such as an MRI or CT scan, can help look for underlying conditions that could be causing

your leg ulcers, such as arterial insufficiency or venous insufficiency.
- A skin biopsy is a procedure in which a small piece of skin is removed and examined under a microscope. This can help to rule out other conditions that may be causing your leg ulcer, such as skin cancer.

Leg Ulcers Risk Factors

Several different factors can increase your risk of developing leg ulcers. These include:

- Age: Older age is a risk factor for leg ulcers because the veins in your legs can become less elastic and more likely to develop valves that are damaged or not functioning properly.
- Obesity: This is a risk factor for leg ulcers because it can put extra pressure on the veins in your legs and make them more likely to develop valves that are damaged or not functioning properly.
- Pregnancy: This is also a risk factor for leg ulcers because it can cause the veins in your legs to enlarge and put extra pressure on the valves.
- Sedentary lifestyle: A sedentary lifestyle is a risk factor for leg ulcers because it can cause the veins in your legs to become more sluggish and more likely to develop valves that are damaged or not functioning properly.

- Smoking: This is a risk factor for leg ulcers because it can damage the veins in your legs and make them more likely to develop valves that are damaged or not functioning properly.
- Diabetes: Diabetes is a risk factor for leg ulcers because it can cause neuropathy, which can lead to nerve damage and decreased blood flow to the legs.
- Venous insufficiency: Venous insufficiency is a risk factor for leg ulcers because it can cause the veins in your legs to not function properly or become damaged, leading to the pooling of blood and increased pressure on the valves.
- Arterial insufficiency: Arterial insufficiency is a risk factor for leg ulcers because it can cause decreased blood flow to the legs.
- Neuropathy: Neuropathy is a risk factor for leg ulcers because it can cause nerve damage and decreased blood flow to the legs.
- Pressure ulcers: Pressure ulcers are a risk factor for leg ulcers because they can lead to decreased blood flow to the legs.
- Infection: Infection is a risk factor for leg ulcers because it can cause inflammation and damage to the veins in your legs.

What Are the Complications of Leg Ulcers?

Wounds on the legs can take a long time to heal and can lead to several complications. If not treated promptly and properly, leg ulcers can be extremely serious and even life-threatening.

Infection

Leg ulcers can become infected, which can lead to sepsis, a potentially life-threatening condition.

Gangrene

Gangrene is a condition in which the tissue in the legs dies due to a lack of blood flow. This can lead to amputation.

Venous insufficiency

Venous insufficiency is a condition in which the veins in your legs are not able to pump blood back to your heart properly. This can lead to swelling, pain, and ulcers.

Arterial insufficiency

Arterial insufficiency is a condition in which the arteries in your legs are not able to provide enough blood flow. This can lead to pain, ulcers, and gangrene.

Deep vein thrombosis

Deep vein thrombosis is a condition in which a blood clot forms in the veins of your legs. This can lead to pain, swelling, and an increased risk of pulmonary embolism, a potentially life-threatening condition.

Lymphedema

Lymphedema is a condition in which fluid builds up in the tissues of your legs. This can lead to pain, swelling, and an increased risk of infection.

Skin cancer

Leg ulcers can increase your risk of developing skin cancer.

How Can You Prevent Leg Ulcers?

Leg ulcers are a common problem, particularly for older adults. The good news is that there are a few things you can do to prevent them.

Control your diabetes: If you have diabetes, it is important to control your blood sugar levels. High blood sugar levels can damage the veins and arteries in your legs and make them more likely to develop ulcers.

Treat venous insufficiency: If you have venous insufficiency, it is important to receive treatment. Treatment may include wearing compression stockings and elevating your legs.

Treat arterial insufficiency: If you have arterial insufficiency, it is important to receive treatment. Treatment may include medications, surgery, and lifestyle changes.

Quit smoking: If you smoke, quitting is important for preventing leg ulcers. Smoking can damage the veins in your legs and make them more likely to develop valves that are damaged or not functioning properly.

Exercise: Exercise is important for people with diabetes, venous insufficiency, and arterial insufficiency. Exercise can help to improve blood flow and decrease swelling.

Wear compression stockings: Wearing compression stockings can help to decrease swelling and improve blood flow.

Manage your weight: If you are overweight, losing weight can help to decrease the pressure on your legs and reduce your risk of developing leg ulcers.

Avoid standing or sitting for long periods: If you must stand or sit for long periods, take breaks and elevate your legs.

Avoid crossing your legs: Crossing your legs can reduce blood flow to your legs and increase your risk of developing leg ulcers.

Inspect your legs daily: Inspect your legs daily for any changes.

Different Treatments for Leg Ulcers

Traditional Treatments

Leg ulcers are a common problem, especially among the elderly. They can be caused by several factors, including circulatory problems, diabetes, and injuries. They are often treated with compression therapy and special bandages. Surgery may also be necessary in some cases.

Compression therapy

Compression therapy is a treatment in which compression bandages or stockings are used to apply pressure to the legs. This can help to decrease swelling and improve blood flow.

Wound care

Wound care is a treatment in which the ulcer is cleaned and dressed. This can help to prevent infection and promote healing.

Surgery

Surgery may be necessary in some cases to treat underlying conditions that are causing leg ulcers, such as arterial insufficiency or venous insufficiency.

Medications

Medications may be necessary in some cases to treat underlying conditions that are causing leg ulcers, such as diabetes or an infection.

Natural Treatments

Leg ulcers are a common problem, and can be quite difficult to manage. Fortunately, there are many natural ways to treat leg ulcers, which can often be more effective than traditional treatments.

Diet

A healthy diet is important for people with leg ulcers. Eating foods that are high in fiber can help to decrease swelling and improve blood flow. Drinking plenty of fluids can also help to keep the legs hydrated and prevent constipation, which can worsen leg ulcers.

Exercise

For people suffering from leg ulcers, exercise is an important part of treatment. Exercise helps to improve blood flow and decrease swelling. This can speed up the healing process and prevent new ulcers from forming.

Walking is a particularly good exercise for people with leg ulcers, as it is low-impact and easy on the joints. However, any type of moderate-intensity exercise can be beneficial.

It is important to consult with a doctor before starting an exercise program, as some exercises may aggravate the condition. With the doctor's approval, however, exercise can be an effective treatment for leg ulcers.

Quit smoking

If you smoke, quitting is important for healing leg ulcers. Smoking can damage the veins in your legs and make them more likely to develop valves that are damaged or not functioning properly.

Ways to Manage Leg Ulcers

Home Therapy

If you're suffering from leg ulcers, you know how painful and frustrating they can be. But there is hope! Several home remedies are effective in managing leg ulcers. From aloe vera to turmeric, there's sure to be a home remedy that can help you find relief from your leg ulcers.

Aloe vera

Aloe vera is a well-known home cure for leg ulcers. The plant comprises a variety of chemicals that have been proven to help wounds heal. Aloe vera gel can be directly applied to the leg ulcer and left to dry naturally.

Turmeric

Turmeric is another popular home remedy for leg ulcers. The spice contains a compound called curcumin, which has powerful anti-inflammatory and antioxidant properties. Turmeric can be taken orally in capsule form or applied topically to the leg ulcer.

Vinegar

Vinegar is another simple home remedy that can be used to treat leg ulcers. Vinegar contains acetic acid, which is effective in killing bacteria and promoting healing. Vinegar can be applied directly to the leg ulcer with a cotton ball or added to a warm bath and soaked for 20 minutes.

Honey

Honey is a natural antibacterial and has been used to treat wounds for centuries. Honey can be applied directly to the leg ulcer or mixed with turmeric to create a paste.

There are a variety of home remedies that can be used to effectively treat leg ulcers. Some of these are coconut oil, lavender oil, and calendula. If you're suffering from leg ulcers, try one of these home remedies and see if it provides you with relief.

Diet

If you suffer from leg ulcers, you may be interested in learning about the recommended diet for venous insufficiency. According to the Physicians Vein Clinics website, certain foods can help improve your condition.

Foods to Eat

High-fiber foods: A diet rich in high-fiber foods, such as fruits and vegetables, can help improve your leg ulcer condition by promoting regularity and helping to reduce constipation. Additionally, fiber has been shown to reduce inflammation in the body, which can worsen leg ulcer symptoms. For these reasons, incorporating high-fiber foods into your diet may help improve your leg ulcer condition.

Examples of high-fiber fruits and vegetables are:

- raspberries
- blackberries
- oranges
- prunes
- broccoli
- spinach
- kale

Potassium-enriched foods: Foods that are rich in potassium, such as bananas, can help to reduce leg swelling. Potassium helps to regulate fluid balance in the body and can also help to reduce inflammation.

Examples of potassium-enriched foods are:

- bananas
- cantaloupe
- honeydew melon
- mangoes
- oranges
- papayas

Vitamin C-rich foods: Vitamin C is a powerful antioxidant that can help to reduce inflammation and promote healing. Foods that are rich in vitamin C, such as strawberries, oranges, and bell peppers, can help improve your leg ulcer condition.

Examples of Vitamin C-rich foods are:

- strawberries
- oranges
- bell peppers
- dark leafy greens
- broccoli
- tomatoes

Flavonoid-enriched foods: One way to help promote healing and reduce the risk of complications is to consume flavonoid-rich foods. Flavonoids are antioxidants that can help to reduce inflammation and improve circulation. leg ulcers often occur in people who have poor circulation, so improving circulation can help heal leg ulcers. In addition, flavonoids can help to protect against infection and keep the skin healthy.

Examples of flavonoid-enriched foods are:

- dark chocolate
- red wine
- berries
- onions

- celery

Water: Drinking plenty of water is important for overall health, but it can also help to reduce leg swelling. When your body is well-hydrated, it can more easily circulate blood and reduce fluid retention.

Foods to Avoid

Processed foods/Salty foods: When your body breaks down these foods, they release compounds that cause inflammation. This can worsen the symptoms of leg ulcers, as well as make it harder for them to heal.

In addition, processed foods and foods high in salt can cause your body to retain fluid. This leads to swelling, which can put added pressure on leg ulcers and make them more difficult to heal. If you suffer from leg ulcers, it's best to avoid these foods as much as possible.

Caffeine: Caffeine is a diuretic, which means it causes the body to lose water. This can lead to dehydration, which can make leg ulcer symptoms worse. Caffeine is also a stimulant, which can increase heart rate and blood pressure. These effects can aggravate leg ulcer symptoms.

Alcohol: Alcohol consumption can lead to several negative health consequences, including dehydration and inflammation. For people who suffer from leg ulcers, these effects can be especially problematic. Alcohol dehydrates the body by causing it to lose fluids more quickly than it can replace them. This can lead to impaired organ function and an increased risk of infection.

Additionally, alcohol consumption can cause inflammation, which can worsen leg ulcers and delay healing. For these reasons, it is generally advisable for people with leg ulcers to avoid alcohol or drink in moderation.

By following these dietary guidelines, you can help improve your leg ulcer condition and prevent further complications. Eating a healthy diet is an important part of managing your leg ulcers, so talk to your doctor or dietitian if you have any questions.

7-Day Sample Meal Plan

Here is a sample meal plan made for a week that you can either follow or modify accordingly. The meals listed below are lifted from the sample recipes included in this guide. The purpose of creating a meal plan is to help you watch what you are about to consume and make sure you're meeting your daily nutrition needs.

7-Day Sample Meal Plan

Meal	Breakfast	Lunch	Dinner
Day 1	Macrobiotic Apple and Oats Porridge	No-Fuss Tuna Casserole	Kale Fried Rice

Day 2	Grilled Eggplant	Apple in Pork Chops	Tangy Lemon Fish
Day 3	Nut Truffle	Chicken Pot Pie	Low FODMAP Burger
Day 4	Vietnamese Early Rush Baguette	Roasted Chicken Thighs	Grilled Tuna
Day 5	Grilled Eggplant	Kale Fried Rice	Steamed Cauliflower and Curried Shrimp
Day 6	Low FODMAP Burger	Tangy Lemon Fish	Grilled Tuna
Day 7	Vegan Tiramisu	Blackened Shrimp	Apple in Pork Chops

Sample Recipes

No-Fuss Tuna Casserole

Ingredients:

- 1-5 oz. can tuna, drained
- 1 can cream of chicken soup, condensed
- 3 cups macaroni, cooked
- 1-1/2 cups fried onions
- 1 cup Cheddar cheese, shredded

Instructions:

1. Preheat the oven to 350°F.
2. Prepare a 9x13-inch baking dish. Use that to mix the macaroni, tuna, and soup. Top it with cheese.
3. Bake for 25 minutes or until the casserole is bubbly.
4. Sprinkle it with fried onions. Put back in the oven and leave for 5 more minutes.
5. Serve and enjoy while hot.

Tangy Lemon Fish

Ingredients:

- 200 g. Gurnard fresh fish fillets
- 3 tbsp. butter
- 1 tbsp. fresh lemon juice
- 1/4 cup fine almond flour
- 1 tsp. dried dill
- 1 tsp. dried chives
- 1 tsp. onion powder
- 1/2 tsp. garlic powder
- salt
- pepper

Instructions:

1. On a large plate or tray, combine dill, almond flour, and spices. Mix until well combined.
2. Dredge each fillet one at a time into the flour mix. Turn the fillet around until fully coated, and then transfer it to a clean plate or tray. This may be refrigerated until ready to cook.
3. Place a large pan over medium-high heat.
4. Combine halves of butter and lemon juice. Swirl the pan to mix, and lift occasionally to avoid burning the butter.
5. Allow the fish to cook for about 3 minutes.

6. Let the fish absorb all the lemony-butter mixture. Cook on low heat to avoid drying out the pan.
7. Add the remaining lemon juice and butter to the pan.
8. Turn the fish to cook the other side for 3 minutes more. Swirl around the pan to fully coat it with the juice.
9. Wait until it turns golden brown and the fish is cooked through.
10. Serve with buttered vegetables.

Vietnamese Early Rush Baguette

Ingredients:

For the tofu marinade:

- 2 tbsp. maple syrup
- 3 tbsp. lime juice
- 2 tbsp. coconut aminos
- 1 block extra-firm tofu
- 1 clove garlic
- 1 tbsp. smoked paprika

For the sandwich:

- 2 scallions
- 1/2 cup vegan mayo
- 4 sliced fresh baguettes
- 1/8 cup fresh cilantro

For the pickles:

- 2 small carrots, julienned
- 1 small radish, julienned
- 1/4 cup of rice vinegar
- 1/4 cup white wine vinegar
- salt, to taste
- turmeric, to taste

Instructions:

For the tofu:

1. Drain excess liquid from the tofu. Slice into baguette-sized portions and place in a medium-sized bowl
2. Add the ingredients for the marinade. Set aside for 20 minutes.
3. Transfer marinated tofu slices to a grilling pan.
4. Grill for about 4 minutes per side.
5. Prepare a bottle of vegan mayo; set it aside for later.

For the pickles:

1. In a medium-sized bowl, add salt and turmeric.
2. Add radish and julienned carrots. Allow marinating for 15 minutes or longer.
3. Prepare the baguettes and spread vegan mayo on top.
4. Assemble the hearty breakfast veggie baguette by layering the pickled vegetables and tofu slices.
5. Serve on a plate and top with extra tomato slices and cilantro for garnishing.

Macrobiotic Apple and Oats Porridge

Ingredients:

- 1 cup oats
- water
- 5 cups apples, cubed
- Stevia sweetener, to taste
- cardamom
- juice from 1 pc lemon
- raisins, for toppings

Instructions:

1. Cook oats in a small pan until done.
2. Add the ingredients and mix to combine on medium to low heat.
3. As the apples soften, take off the heat.
4. Serve with raisins on top of the oats.

Vegan Tiramisu

Ingredients:

Cake:

- 1 cup, less than 2 tbsp. oat flour
- 2-1/2 tbsp. corn starch
- 1/4 cup organic cane sugar
- 1/2 cup non-dairy milk
- 2 tbsp. almond milk yogurt
- 1 tsp. vanilla extract
- 2 tsp. baking powder

Pudding:

- 8 pitted Medjool dates
- 2 cups non-dairy milk
- 3 tbsp. corn starch
- 2 tsp. vanilla extract
- 1 tbsp. lemon juice
- 1 tbsp. cacao powder
- 1/2 cup brewed coffee or Teeccino

Instructions:

To make the cake:

1. Preheat the oven to 350°F.
2. Sift the oat flour, baking powder, and cornstarch into a mixing bowl.

3. Add the rest of the ingredients and whisk till smooth.
4. Pour a shallow layer of cake into the bottom of an 8×8" square pan lined with parchment paper.
5. Bake for 10-11 minutes until the center bounces back when touched.
6. Set aside to cool.

To make the pudding:

1. Blend all the ingredients on high till smooth.
2. Pour into a large heat-safe bowl.
3. Microwave on high for a minute. Whisk. Then microwave for another minute on high until thickened.
4. Let it cool with a piece of plastic wrap on top so it doesn't form that weird layer.

To assemble:

1. After cooling down, slice the cake into cubes.
2. Dip each cube into the coffee.
3. Layer them on the bottom of the glass.
4. Layer the pudding on top and dust with cacao powder.

Nut Truffle

Ingredients:

- 1 cup raw almonds
- 1-2 cups pinto beans, cooked or drained from a can
- 3 tbsp. syrup, agave or pure maple
- 1/4 cup cocoa, dark for intense flavor
- 2 tbsp. oil
- 1 cup semi-sweet chocolate chips

Instructions:

1. Using a food processor, chop almonds.
2. Add the beans, 2 tbsp. syrup, and cocoa. Process again.
3. Add the leftover syrup and process for the last time.
4. Roll the mixture into balls. Refrigerate after.
5. Make the chocolate dip by combining oil and semi-sweet chocolate chips. Mix continuously until melted.
6. Dip and cover the balls in the chocolate.
7. Place on wax paper and leave to chill.
8. When the truffles are firm, it is ready to be served.

Blackened Shrimp

Ingredients:

- 1/2 lb. shrimp, deveined and peeled
- 2 tbsp. blackening seasoning
- 1 lemon, juice only
- 1 tsp. olive oil

Seasoning:

- 1 tbsp. sea salt, coarse
- 1 tbsp. black pepper
- 2-1/2 tbsp. paprika
- 1 tbsp. onion powder
- 1 tbsp. cayenne pepper
- 2 tbsp. garlic powder
- 1 tbsp. thyme, dried
- 1 tbsp. oregano, dried

Instructions:

1. In a bowl, mix the seasoning ingredients. Store in a container until use.
2. In a bowl, add the shrimp. Toss with the seasoning and lemon juice.
3. In a non-stick skillet, heat oil on medium-high. Add the shrimp and cook for 2 to 3 minutes on each side.
4. Serve and enjoy while hot.

Grilled Tuna

Ingredients:

- tuna
- 4 tbsp. lemon juice
- 2 cloves garlic, minced
- salt
- pepper

Instructions:

1. Marinate tuna with garlic and lemon juice.
2. Season with salt and pepper.
3. Grill for 8-10 minutes.
4. Add more fresh ground pepper upon serving.
5. Serve and enjoy while hot.

Chicken Pot Pie

Ingredients:

For the chicken filling:

- 1.5 lb. organic chicken breasts, cut into half-inch cubes
- 1 tbsp. butter
- 4 oz. yellow onion, finely chopped
- 1 clove garlic, crushed
- 1/4 cup carrots, finely diced
- 1/2 tsp. dried thyme
- 1 cup chicken broth, low sodium
- 1 tbsp. white wine vinegar
- 1/4 cup peas, fresh or frozen
- 1/4–1/2 tsp. sea salt
- 1/2 cup heavy cream
- 1/4 tsp. freshly ground black pepper

For the topping:

- 1 cup superfine almond flour
- 1/2 tsp. xanthan gum
- 1 tbsp. ground flax seeds
- 1 tsp. baking powder
- 2 tbsp. butter, cut into large chunks
- 1/4 tsp. sea salt
- 2 tbsp. sour cream
- 1 egg white

Instructions:

1. Preheat the oven to 400°F.
2. Grease a 9" round baking pan.

For the chicken filling:

1. Melt butter on a large skillet over medium-high heat.
2. Add the diced chicken to the pan.
3. Stir chicken occasionally, until they begin to turn brown on all sides but are not yet cooked throughout.
4. Add onion and carrots to the skillet.
5. Sprinkle the mixture lightly with salt and pepper. Turn heat to medium-low.
6. Cook, stirring occasionally until the onions begin to brown at the edges but are not yet tender.
7. Stir in garlic and dried thyme. Cook for one minute, stirring constantly.
8. Stir in vinegar, scraping up browned bits. When the vinegar has almost completely evaporated, stir in broth.
9. Adjust heat to medium-high and wait for the broth to simmer, while stirring occasionally, for about 15-20 minutes, or until it thickens.
10. Add heavy cream and peas when the broth has thickened.
11. Reduce heat and allow the broth to simmer until the mixture is thick and similar to gravy.
12. Season with salt and pepper, if necessary.

For the topping:

1. Whisk together the almond flour, xanthan gum, ground flax seeds, baking powder, and salt.
2. Use a pastry blender to cut the butter into the dry ingredients.
3. Whisk the egg white and the sour cream together in a separate bowl.
4. Stir the sour cream mixture into the dry ingredients.
5. Gather the mixture into a ball and place it on a piece of parchment paper or a counter dusted with almond flour.
6. Press or roll dough into a circle about 8 inches in diameter.

Assembly:

1. Transfer the chicken filling to the baking dish prepared beforehand.
2. Carefully place the biscuit dough over the filling.
3. Bake until the topping has turned brown, about 10-12 minutes.

Apple in Pork Chops

Ingredients:

- 1 tbsp. onion, chopped
- 1/4 cup celery, chopped
- 2 cups apples, chopped
- 2 tsp. fresh parsley, chopped
- 3 cups bread crumbs, fresh
- 6 pcs. thick pork chops, 1.25"
- 1 tbsp. vegetable oil
- 1/4 cup butter
- 1/4 tsp. + more salt
- pepper

Instructions:

1. Preheat the oven to 350°F.
2. Heat butter in a large skillet, and saute onion. Remove from heat.
3. Mix in apples, bread crumbs, celery, parsley, and 1/4 teaspoon salt. Set aside the apple mixture
4. Cut open a side of the pork chop to create a pocket.
5. Season it with salt and pepper, both in the pocket and the entire pork chop.
6. Add a spoonful of apple mixture into the pockets. Don't stuff it in.
7. Heat oil in a skillet over medium-high heat. Cook chops until both sides are brown.

8. Transfer to a 9x13-inch baking dish that is ungreased. Cover with aluminum foil.
9. Bake in the oven for half an hour.
10. Remove the foil and bake for another half hour or until the juices look clear.

Kale Fried Rice

Ingredients:

- 2 tbsp. coconut oil
- 2 whole eggs
- 2 large garlic cloves, minced
- 3 large green onions, thinly sliced
- 1 cup carrots, cut into matchsticks
- 1 cup Brussels sprouts, diced
- 1 medium bunch of kale, ribs removed and the leaves shredded
- 2 cups brown rice, cooked and cooled
- 1/4 tsp. Himalayan salt
- 1/4 cup lemon balm leaves, diced
- 3/4 cups shredded coconut, unsweetened variety
- fresh cilantro, for garnishing

Instructions:

1. Heat a teaspoon of oil in a large skillet over medium-high heat.
2. Pour in the egg mixture.
3. Cook the eggs while occasionally stirring.
4. Remove from the pan and set aside.
5. Pour another teaspoon of coconut oil into the pan, along with Brussels sprouts, carrots, garlic, and green onions.
6. Stir now and then until the vegetables look tender.

7. Add kale and salt.
8. Remove from the pan and put them into where the egg is.
9. Put the remaining coconut oil into the pan. Add in coconut flakes, stirring frequently
10. Add rice and stir it in.
11. Add the egg and vegetable mixture to the pan, as well as the lemon balm leaves.
12. Stir to combine and heat through.
13. Transfer to a serving bowl and garnish with fresh cilantro.
14. Serve and enjoy.

Grilled Eggplant

Ingredients:

- 2 small eggplants or 1 large eggplant, around 1-1/4 to 1-1/12 lb. in total, sliced into half-inch-thick rounds
- 2 tbsp. extra-virgin olive oil
- salt

Instructions:

1. Preheat the grill using the medium-high setting.
2. Toss eggplant slices and olive oil in a bowl.
3. Sprinkle it with salt to taste.
4. Toss ingredients again.
5. Place eggplant slices onto the grill.
6. Turn over to the other side after about 4 minutes, or until charred spots have appeared on the underside.
7. Continue grilling until eggplant slices have become tender.
8. When storing, place into an airtight container once it has cooled down, and then refrigerate. Grilled eggplant can last for up to 4 days in a chilled condition.

Low FODMAP Burger

Ingredients:

- 1-1/4 lbs. ground pork
- 1/4 tsp. allspice
- 1/2 tsp. salt
- 1/2 tsp. white pepper
- 1/2 tsp. ground nutmeg
- 1/2 tsp. caraway seeds
- 1/2 tsp. ground ginger

Instructions:

1. Preheat the grill then prepare the patty.
2. Using a small mixing bowl, stir together the salt, pepper, allspice, nutmeg, and ginger until fully combined.
3. Place the ground in a large mixing bowl and add the spice mixture.
4. Mix thoroughly until spices are evenly distributed to the pork.
5. Make round, flat burger patties using the palm of your hands.
6. Grill the patties and serve with gluten-free buns and mustard sauce.

Roasted Chicken Thighs

Ingredients:

- 12 garlic cloves, unpeeled
- 1 tbsp. avocado oil
- 1 pinch Himalayan pink salt
- 4 chicken thighs with skin
- 1 tsp. Primal Palate super gyro seasoning

Instructions:

1. Pour avocado oil over a medium-sized oven-safe pot.
2. Add the garlic cloves. Sauté over medium heat for 2 to 3 minutes or until the skins begin to brown.
3. Place the chicken in a large skillet over medium-high heat. Sear for about 2 to 3 minutes for each side, starting with the skin side.
4. Combine the chicken with the garlic. Season generously with salt and Primal Palate Super Gyro seasoning.
5. Place the chicken in an oven preheated to 350°F.
6. Bake for one hour while covered.
7. Serve and enjoy.

Steamed Cauliflower and Curried Shrimp

Ingredients:

- 1 whole cauliflower, separated into florets
- 2 tbsp. canola oil
- 2 cloves garlic, minced
- 1 cup sweet peppers, chopped finely
- 1 lb. bay shrimp, pre-cooked
- 1 tsp. curry powder
- 1 tsp. butter
- 3 tbsp. flour
- 1/2 cup fish or vegetable broth
- 2/3 cup milk, low-fat
- 1 tbsp. fresh dill, finely chopped
- 1/4 cup pine nuts, toasted

Instructions:

1. Steam the cauliflower until tender. Set aside.
2. Use a frying pan to sauté the garlic. Add the peppers. Continue cooking until the peppers start to soften.
3. Add the curry powder and the shrimp. Remove pan from heat and set aside.
4. Prepare the roux. Melt the butter. Add the flour and whisk. Heat until the roux becomes light golden brown.

5. Add the milk and broth to the roux gradually. Whisk to incorporate. Stir constantly until the sauce starts to bubble.
6. Add the curried shrimp. Bring the heat down and cook for another 5 minutes.
7. Toss the cauliflower in the shrimp sauce.
8. Transfer to a serving platter. Garnish with dill and pine nuts.

Conclusion

While the exact cause of leg ulcers is often unknown, there are several potential contributing factors, including poor circulation, diabetes, and inflammation. Fortunately, several natural remedies can be used to effectively manage leg ulcers.

For example, eating high-fiber foods, such as fruits and vegetables can help to improve circulation and promote healing. In addition, applying a topical cream or ointment that contains aloe vera or calendula can help to soothe irritated skin and speed up the healing process.

Finally, making some simple diet changes, such as eliminating processed foods and increasing your intake of fiber-rich foods, can also help to reduce inflammation and promote healing. By following these simple tips, you can start managing your leg ulcers naturally and effectively.

FAQ

Q: What are some common symptoms of leg ulcers?

A: Some common symptoms of leg ulcers include pain, itching, and inflammation. The affected area may also be warm to the touch and appear red or discolored.

Q: What is the recommended diet for someone with leg ulcers?

A: The recommended diet for someone with leg ulcers includes high-fiber foods, potassium-rich foods, flavonoid-rich foods, and plenty of water. Processed foods and salty foods should be avoided.

Q: What are some natural remedies for leg ulcers?

A: Some natural remedies for leg ulcers include aloe vera, calendula, and cayenne pepper. These substances can help to soothe irritated skin and speed up the healing process.

Q: Are leg ulcers contagious?

A: No, leg ulcers are not contagious. However, if you have an underlying condition that is causing your leg ulcers, such as diabetes, you may be at risk for other complications. Therefore, it's important to see your doctor for a proper diagnosis and treatment plan.

Q: What are the complications of leg ulcers?

A: If left untreated, leg ulcers can lead to serious complications, such as infection, tissue death, and blood clots. In severe cases, leg amputation may be necessary. Therefore, it's important to see your doctor for proper diagnosis and treatment.

Key Takeaways

- Leg ulcers are painful sores that can occur on the legs.
- The exact cause of leg ulcers is often unknown, but potential causes include poor circulation, diabetes, and inflammation.
- Several natural remedies can be used to effectively manage leg ulcers.
- Making some simple diet changes, such as eliminating processed foods and increasing your intake of fiber-rich foods, can also help to reduce inflammation and promote healing.
- If left untreated, leg ulcers can lead to serious complications, such as infection, tissue death, and blood clots. Therefore, it's important to see your doctor for proper diagnosis and treatment.

If you have any further questions about leg ulcers, be sure to talk to your doctor or healthcare provider.

This article is for informational purposes only and does not constitute medical advice. The information contained herein is not intended to replace a one-on-one relationship with a qualified healthcare professional and is not intended as medical advice.

It is intended as a sharing of knowledge and information from the research and experience of the author. You are encouraged to make your own healthcare decisions based on your research and in partnership with a qualified healthcare professional.

References and Helpful Links

13 home remedies to heal leg ulcers and prevention tips. (2014, May 13). STYLECRAZE. https://www.stylecraze.com/articles/effective-home-remedies-for-leg-ulcers/.

Simion @Yonescat, F. (n.d.). Leg ulcers. Circulation Foundation. Retrieved August 18, 2022, from https://www.circulationfoundation.org.uk/help-advice/veins/leg-ulcers.

The recommended diet for venous insufficiency. (n.d.). Physicians Vein Clinics. Retrieved August 18, 2022, from https://www.physiciansveinclinics.com/blog/recommended-diet-for-venous-insufficiency

Venous leg ulcer. (2017, October 23). NHS.UK. https://www.nhs.uk/conditions/leg-ulcer/.

Wellness library | Cigna. (n.d.). Retrieved August 18, 2022, from https://www.cigna.com/knowledge-center/hw/.

What causes leg ulcers? (2012, July 25). Healthline. https://www.healthline.com/health/leg-ulcers.

www.ingramcontent.com/pod-product-compliance
Lightning Source LLC
LaVergne TN
LVHW012037060526
838201LV00061B/4654